K

OUR HEROES
OF COVID-19

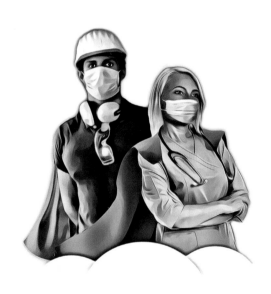

Library and Archives Canada Cataloguing in Publication

Title: Our heroes of COVID-19 / by Phil Riggs ; illustrated by Corey Majeau.
Names: Riggs, Phil, author. | Majeau, Corey, 1985- illustrator.
Identifiers: Canadiana 20200279688 | ISBN 9781989417256 (softcover)
Subjects: LCSH: COVID-19 (Disease)—Juvenile fiction.
Classification: LCC PS8635.I534 O97 2020 | DDC jC813/.6—dc23

Published by Boulder Books
Portugal Cove-St. Philip's, Newfoundland and Labrador
www.boulderbooks.ca

© 2020 Phil Riggs

Layout: Todd Manning
Editor: S.G. Taylor
Copy editor: Iona Bulgin

Printed in Canada

We acknowledge the financial support of the Government of Newfoundland and Labrador through the Department of Tourism, Culture and Recreation.

Newfoundland Labrador

Funded by the Government of Canada   Financé par le gouvernement du Canada

Canada

OUR HEROES
OF COVID-19

STORY BY

Phil Riggs

ILLUSTRATED BY

Corey Majeau

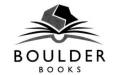

BOULDER
BOOKS

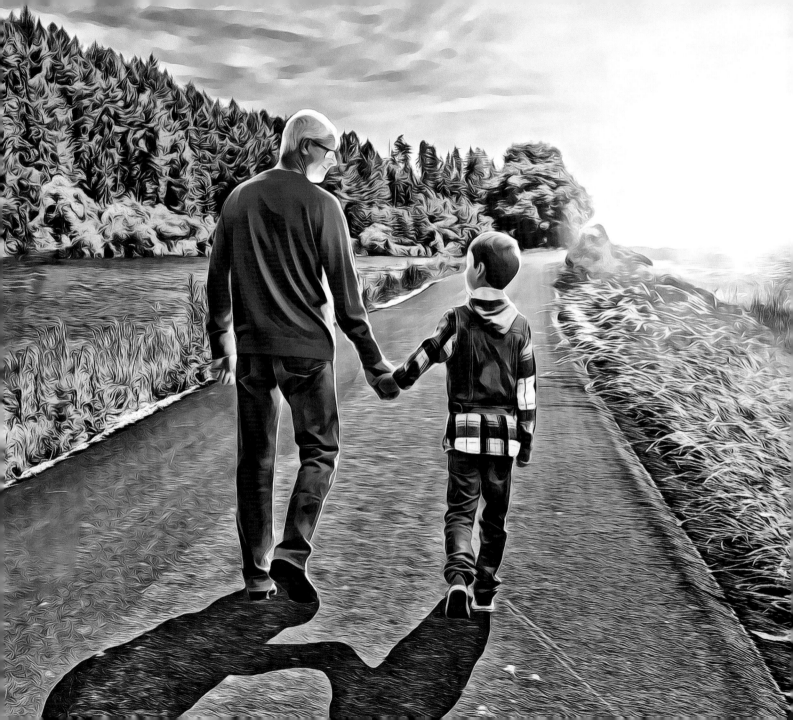

It was a beautiful and bright summer day. A soft breeze was whispering. Squirrels chattered as birds twittered and sang in the trees. The lazy river seemed to gurgle a deep, watery welcome.

Best of all, the COVID-19 shutdown was over—and the sun was smiling down upon it all.

It was a perfect day for Joel and Grandpa to end their social distancing. So, with smiles on their faces, and a brown paper bag filled with duck food, they started their walk to the park.

"Grandpa," said Joel. "I'm so glad we can finally take our walks again!"

"So am I, Joel," Grandpa replied. "Even though we still have to be careful, it is truly a joy to be able to have times like this." Grandpa was silent for a moment, then he said, "You know, Joel, it took quite a few brave people and heroes to make sure it was safe for us to go out again."

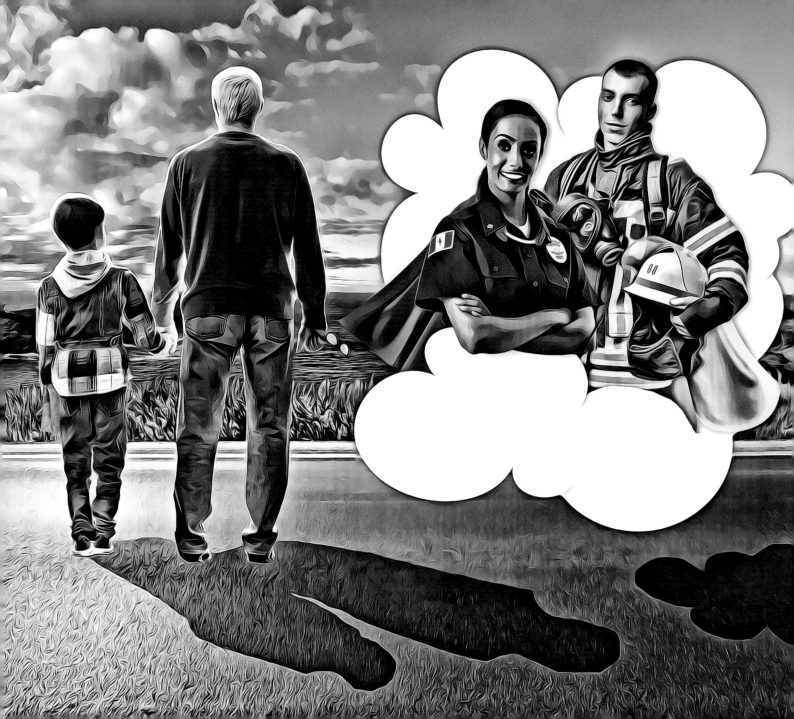

Joel looked up at his grandfather. "Heroes? You mean like firefighters?"

Grandpa nodded. "Yes, indeed. They often put their lives at risk, responding to emergencies. But there were many other heroes, too, during the shutdown. Can you think of any?"

Joel squinted one eye and crinkled his nose as he thought for a moment. "I know!" he said. "Doctors and nurses!"

"You are absolutely right. They help very sick people every day. During the shutdown, they were at even greater risk than normal," Grandpa said. "Do you remember all the people who stood in front of their homes, cheering and clapping as the healthcare workers drove by?"

"Yes, Grandpa!" said Joel. "I cheered for them too!"

"So did I, my boy. It was wonderful to see people supporting one another like that," said Grandpa. "Can you think of any other heroes, Joel?"

Joel squinted one eye and crinkled his nose again, as he thought ...

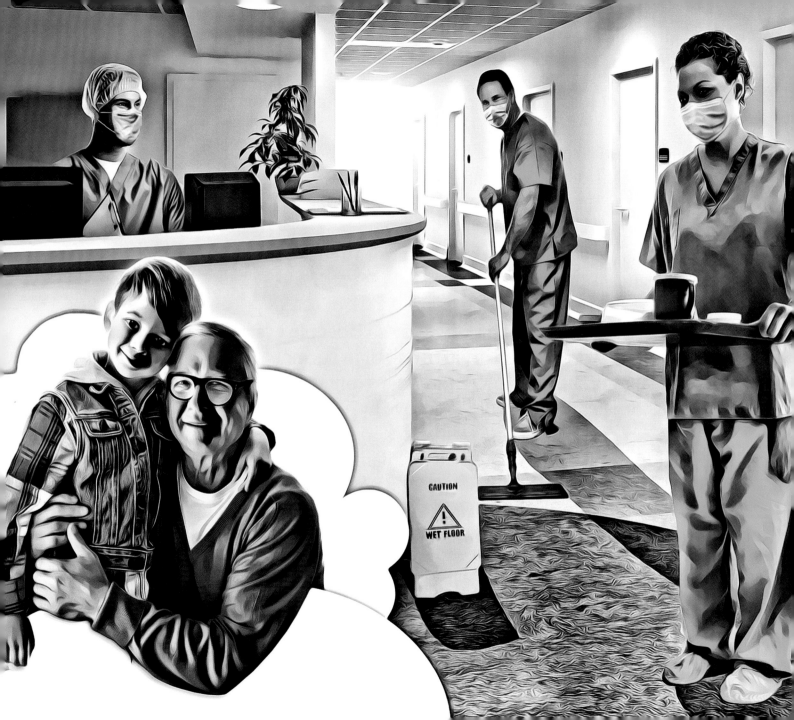

"Our neighbour, Mr. Miller, is a janitor at the hospital. And Mrs. Miller works there in an office," Joel said. "Are *all* the people who work in hospitals heroes, Grandpa?"

"Well, what do you think?" Grandpa asked.

"Hmmm," Joel said. "I think they are very, very brave because they could have gotten the virus, too."

"You're so right. They are essential workers, doing jobs that have to be done," Grandpa continued. "And what about police officers, ambulance drivers, and paramedics?"

"Oh, I know this!" said Joel. "They're called First, um, First Responders! Because they're the first to come help in emergencies!"

Grandpa smiled and squeezed his grandson's hand. "You're very smart!" he said. "First Responders are heroes every day—but especially during COVID-19."

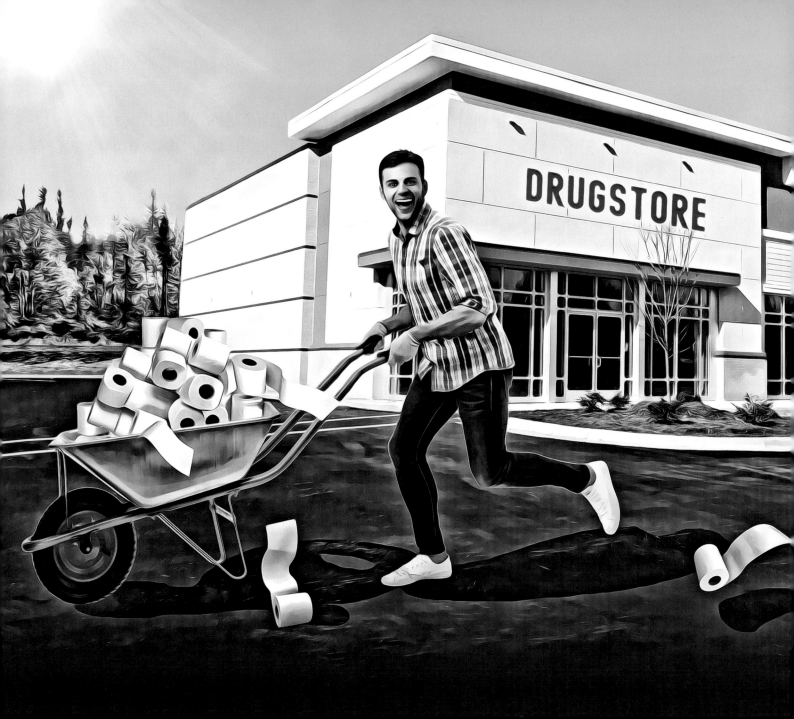

As the neighbourhood drugstore came into view, Grandpa said, "You know, Joel, we depend quite a lot on pharmacy workers too. They had to keep working during the shutdown so that we could get the medicine, vitamins, and other things we need to stay healthy."

"Like when Mommy had to get my cough medicine!" said Joel. "Grandpa, what about people who work in all the other stores?"

"Good thinking," said Grandpa. "Shops of all kinds have to serve many people every day. Those workers were very brave too. Their work is important because so many people need *so* many different things."

"Like milk, bread, bananas, and butter," said Joel. Then he grinned and said, "And lots and lots of toilet paper!"

"Oh yes! I don't think we'll *ever* forget that!" replied Grandpa. They laughed as they walked along, remembering the great toilet paper hunt of 2020.

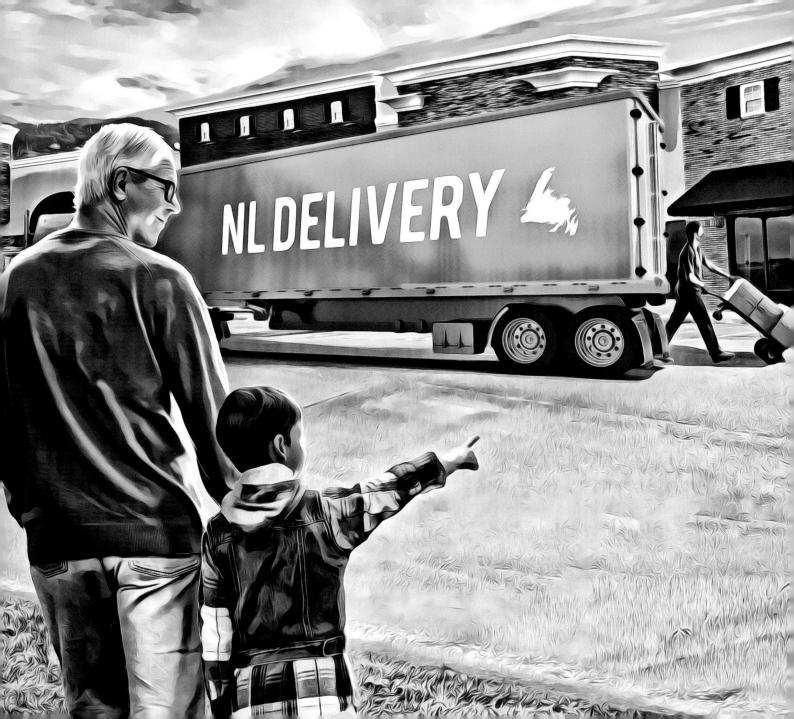

Suddenly, they heard a loud rumble. A big, blue truck appeared and turned toward the supermarket across the street. Joel watched the driver backing up and heard the loud *Pssssssshhhhhh!* of the air brakes.

"What about truck drivers?" asked Grandpa. "Do you think they might be heroes?"

Joel squinted one eye and crinkled his nose again. "Ummm." He wasn't sure. He had not thought about that before.

Grandpa said, "Well, think about all the things they bring us. Not only groceries, but all the other things too, like shoes, clothing, phones, soap ..."

"And ice cream and duck food!" added Joel, shaking the little brown bag.

"Yes, even ice cream and duck food," said Grandpa. "Most things couldn't get here without truck drivers. During the shutdown, they had to keep going, bringing it all from far away."

"So, no ice cream without truck drivers?" asked Joel. "Boy, I'm really glad we have truck drivers."

"So am I," said Grandpa. "Speaking of ice cream, would you like one?"

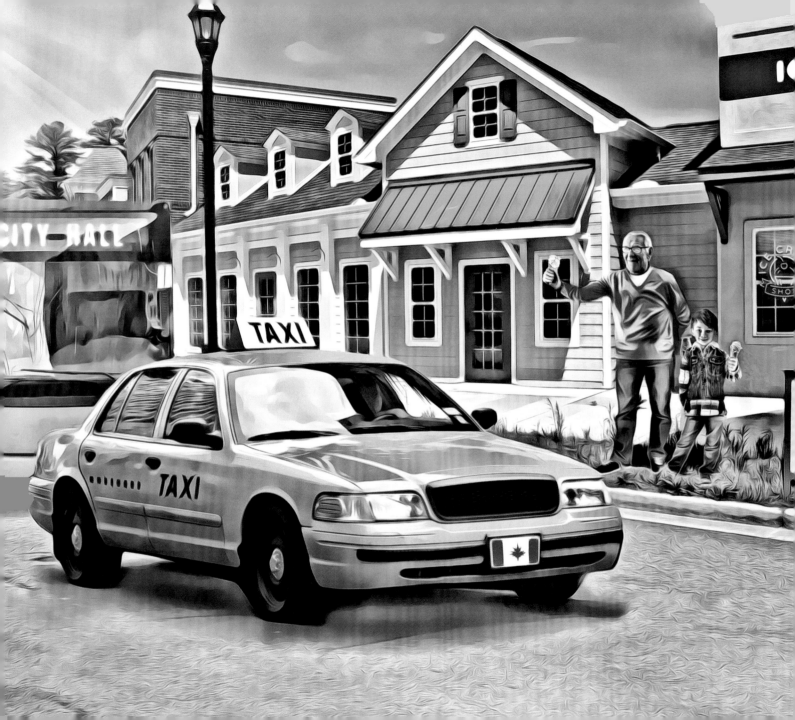

Joel looked up to see a small store with a big ice cream sign in the window. Joel *loved* ice cream—especially strawberry! They went inside and a nice lady put on a pair of thin gloves, then handed them two yummy, pink cones. They walked along enjoying their treats as cars, trucks, taxis, and buses passed by. Then, Joel asked, "Grandpa, what about bus drivers and taxi drivers?"

Grandpa nodded. "Yes, they were brave and worked through the shutdown too, helping people get where they needed to go."

"And, Grandpa, do you know that some people needed help getting food?"

Grandpa nodded. "Yes, my lad. Many folks helped by sending groceries and other important things to food banks. You know, a lot of people donate to food banks often; but during the shutdown, even more was needed. And many kind people responded."

As they finished their ice cream, Grandpa said, "Kindness is one of the most important things in the world, Joel. I hope you always remember to be kind."

"Oh, I will," said Joel, nodding. "And you too, Grandpa." That made Grandpa smile.

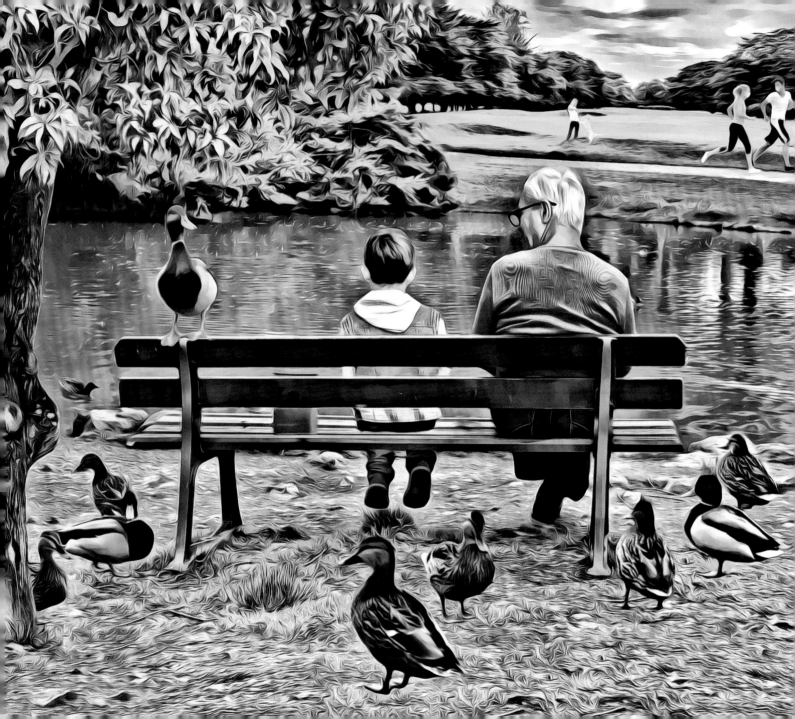

As the pair arrived at the park, dozens of squawking ducks came rushing up to greet them, flapping their wings, waddling and honking all the way. Grandfather and grandson sat on a bench, feeding the noisy, friendly birds.

The scent of fresh-cut grass filled the air. All around, people were walking and jogging. An elderly couple wearing masks sat together, holding hands. A short distance away, children were riding bikes and playing fetch with an excited puppy. Nearby, a busy bumblebee gathered pollen from a bright yellow flower, then happily buzzed away.

Joel and Grandpa were so grateful that the COVID-19 shutdown was over that they both let out a big sigh of contentment at the same time. They giggled about that. After a moment, Joel said, "I hope we never, ever have any more shutdowns, Grandpa."

Grandpa gave Joel a big hug. "So do I, my boy. And if we all cooperate by doing things like washing our hands often, keeping a reasonable distance from people we don't know, and covering our faces if we're in a busy place, we'll have a much better chance of it never being that bad again."

"That sounds smart to me," said Joel happily.

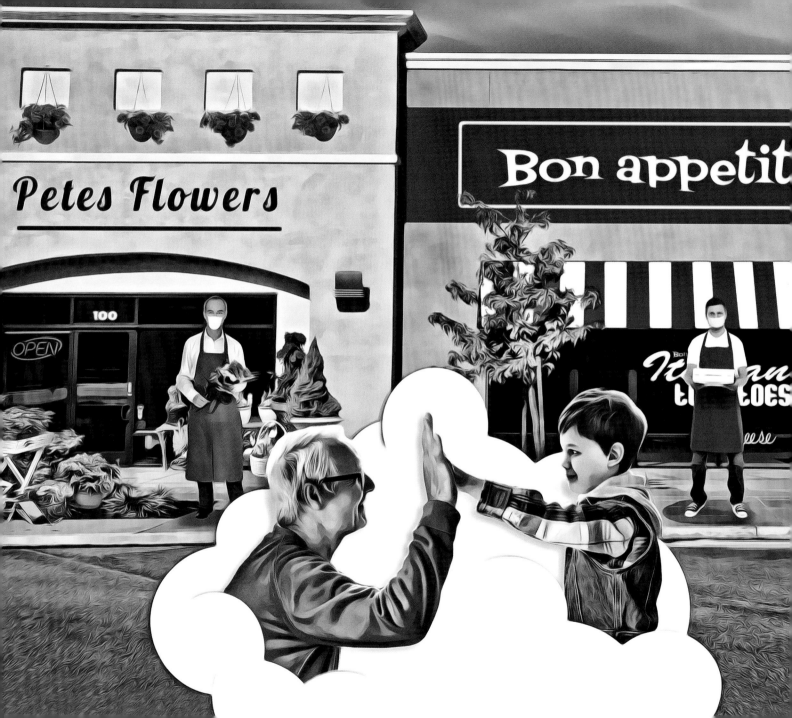

As Grandpa cleaned his eyeglasses, he said, "COVID-19 has been very difficult for everyone. But, you know what? Even in the darkest of times there's a bright light shining in the hearts of good people. So many random acts of kindness. Do you know what I'm talking about, Joel?"

"Yes, I think so, Grandpa," Joel said. "Like the restaurant owners that made free food for people who needed it? And the flower shop owner who gave away flowers?"

"Yes, exactly," Grandpa said. "There are many, many more stories of kindness just like those, Joel. Far too many to count. But each and every one mattered, very much."

Joel looked at Grandpa. "I'm glad there are too many to count," he said.

Grandpa certainly couldn't disagree with that.

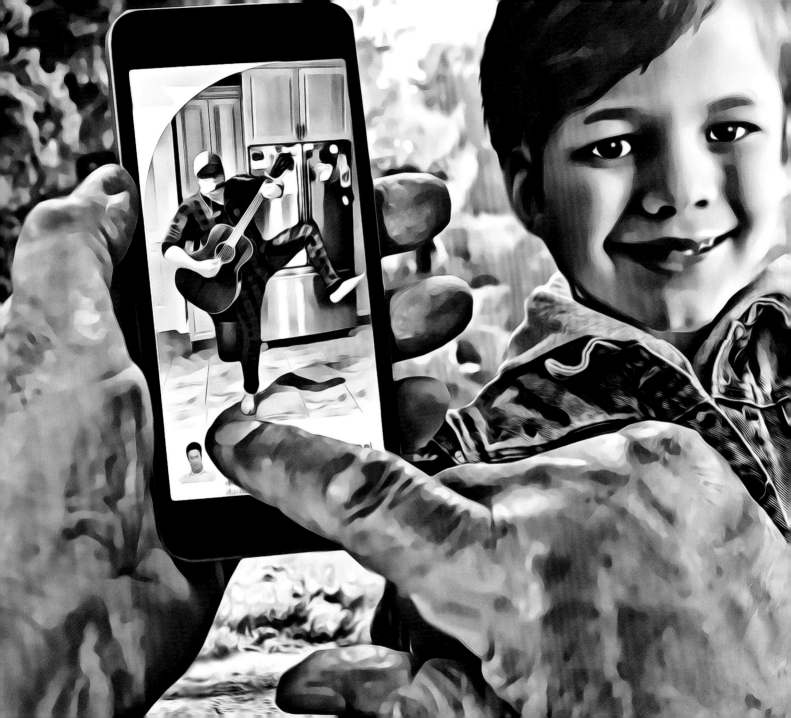

It was getting close to dinnertime, so they started toward home again.

"There was one thing I liked about the shutdown, though, Grandpa," said Joel. "All the videos that people made. They were fun to watch while we were stuck indoors."

"Ah, yes!" said Grandpa. "And all the singers and musicians who shared songs with us on the Internet."

"And the people who dressed up as lions, bears, and other animals to make us laugh!" said Joel. "Do you remember that, Grandpa?"

"Yes, I sure do," said Grandpa. "And do *you* remember when the Easter Bunny was declared an essential worker?"

"Well, that's because he *is*, Grandpa!" explained Joel.

Grandpa chuckled. He certainly couldn't disagree with that either!

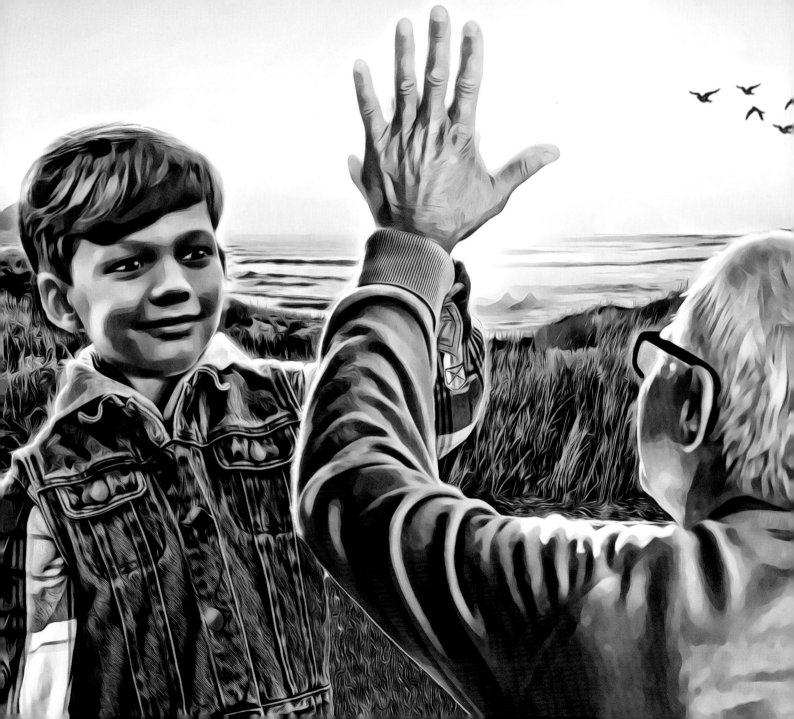

As Joel and Grandpa walked home hand in hand, they were both grateful for the wonderful day they'd had.

Joel was also glad to know that there were so many kind and brave people. Suddenly he said, "Grandpa, I hope *all* the heroes of COVID-19 know we appreciate them."

Grandpa looked at his thoughtful grandson. "I think they do, Joel," he said. "There were so many who worked behind the scenes, quietly doing important jobs that we didn't even know about. They are still heroes to us."

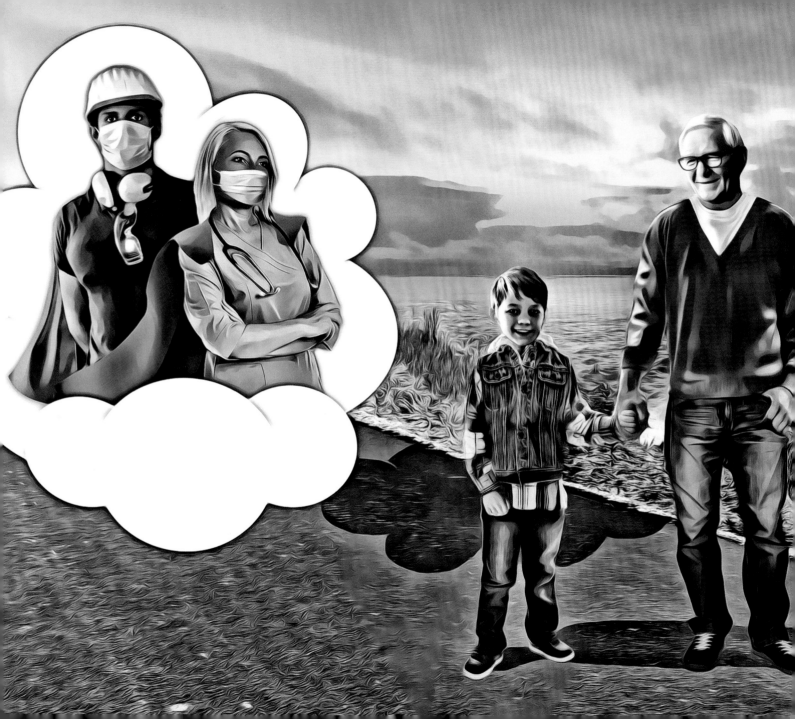

As they neared home, Grandpa said, "I really enjoyed our chat today, Joel."

"Me too, Grandpa," said Joel. Then, once again, he squinted one eye and crinkled his nose.

"I can tell you're thinking about something," said Grandpa.

How did he know that? Joel wondered, but then he said, "Well, what I think is that all those brave people aren't really heroes."

"Really, Joel?" said Grandpa, quite shocked. "Why do you say that?"

"Because I think they're *superheroes*!" exclaimed Joel, in his best superhero voice.

"You know, what, Joel?" Grandpa chuckled. "That's what I think too."

Now share your experiences with COVID-19 by drawing pictures or writing stories.

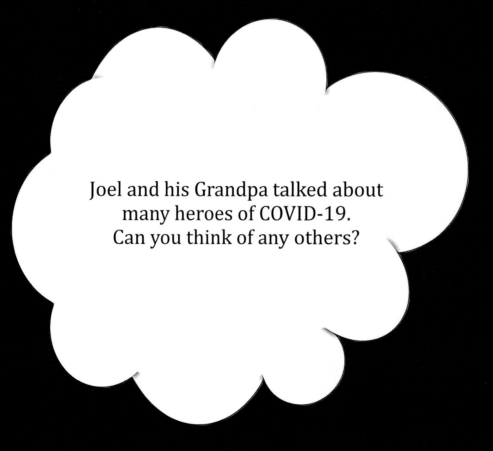

Joel and his Grandpa talked about
many heroes of COVID-19.
Can you think of any others?

What were some of the fun things you did while you had to stay home?

What did you miss the most during the COVID-19 shutdown?

How did your life change during the shutdown?

Draw a picture or tell a story about people doing acts of kindness.

DID YOU KNOW?

In 2019, a new worldwide virus, named COVID-19, appeared and made many people sick. To help stop the virus from spreading, most businesses and schools were shut down and people had to stay safe at home with their families. Everyone had to practice social distancing, and many people wore masks over their noses and mouths whenever they went out in public. Several month later, it became safe enough to start going places and seeing some friends again. And that is when Joel and Grandpa took their lovely walk to the park.

While most of us had to stay at home during the shutdown, not everyone could do that. Many people had to continue working to help keep us all safe and healthy. This is the story of how Joel, Grandpa, and all of us appreciate those brave people—and to remind us that with cooperation and kindness, we can get through any difficult time.